Smoothie Recipes 2021

Delicious Smoothies for Health to Make at Home

License Notes

Table of Contents

Introduction

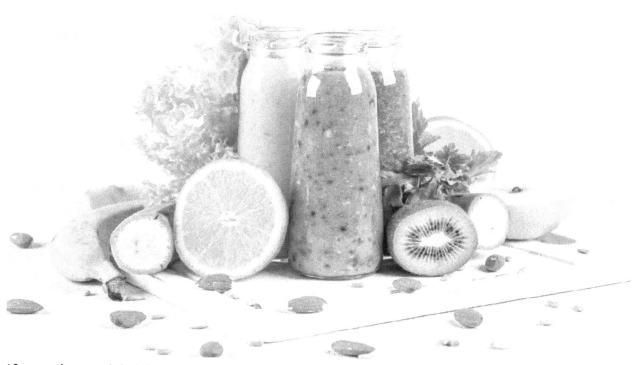

If you love drinking smoothies, then you would enjoy reading this book. The recipes mentioned in this book are just delicious and perfect for living a longer life span.

You can keep your body in a perfect shape with the help of smoothies and regular exercises.

If you are suffering from kidney disease, then we suggest you to avoid drinking green smoothies. You can prepare smoothies in advance and can store them in a fridge for a day or two. Just before serving, don't forget to give it a good stir and enjoy.

With this book, you can choose from plenty of famous smoothie recipes such as Apple Banana Smoothie, Almond Fruit Smoothie, Banana Cinnamon Roll Smoothie, Unicorn Smoothie, Sweet Honeydew Mint Smoothie, Tropical Green Smoothie, Mango Hemp Seeds Green Smoothie, Orange Kale Protein Green Smoothie, Vanilla Matcha Protein Smoothie Recipe, Summer Breezes Smoothie, and many more.

Just tune the pages and show your smoothie skills to your family.

Recipes

Mango Hemp Seeds Green Smoothie

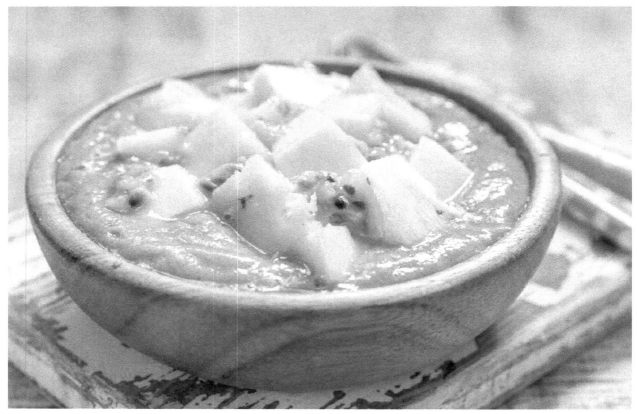

Prep Time: 1 minute

Cooking Time: 1 minute

Servings: 1 person

If you are looking for a green smoothie but don't want to use hemp seeds, then you can sub it with flax seeds. Feel free to use fresh spinach in this smoothie.

Ingredients

- 3 handfuls of fresh baby kale
- ½ cup ripe mango, diced
- 2 tablespoons hemp seeds
- 1 banana, medium-sized
- ½ cup almond milk, unsweetened or any of your favorite milk
- A handful of ice
- 1/8 teaspoon sea salt or pink salt

For Topping:

- A drizzle of pure honey
- Sliced mango
- Red Russian kale sprouts
- Hemp seeds

Directions

Process the ingredients in a blender until completely smooth and creamy.

Pour the prepared smoothie into a large bowl & layer with the toppings such as a drizzle of honey, sliced mango, red Russian kale sprouts and hemp seeds.

Nutritional Value: kcal: 400, Fat: 12 g, Fiber: 10 g, Protein: 19 g

Strawberry Pomegranate Green Smoothie

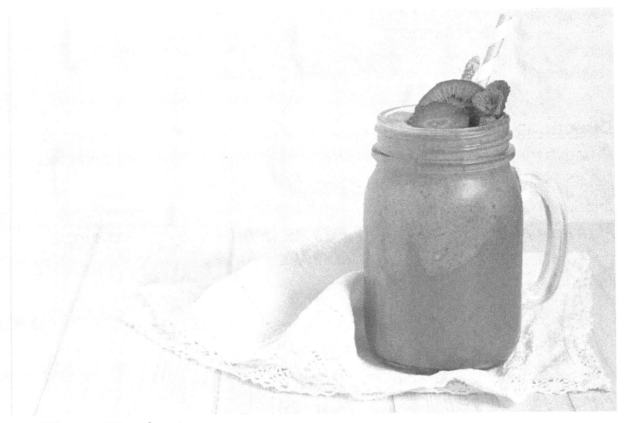

Prep Time: 10 minutes

Cooking Time: 25 minutes

Servings: 6 persons

You would just fall in love with this two colors smoothie. For added nutrition, feel free to add Greek yogurt to this smoothie. Absolutely delicious and healthy!

<u>Ingredients</u>

For Green Layer:

- ¼ cup pomegranate arils
- 1 cup spinach, fresh
- ¼ cup coconut water, cream skimmed
- ½ banana, frozen

For Pink Layer:

- 1 cup strawberries, fresh or frozen
- ½ cup coconut water, cream skimmed
- 1 medium-sized banana, frozen

Directions

Create the pink layer first by blending all of the ingredients together in a blender, on high power until smooth, set aside.

Wipe out your blender and then, create the green layer following the same steps mentioned above.

Once done, pour the pink smoothie first into a large glass and then carefully pour the green one, preferably in a very slow and steady stream, don't stir. Serve as it is and enjoy.

Nutritional Value: kcal: 280, Fat: 2 g, Fiber: 11 g, Protein: 4.9 g

Snickerdoodle Green Smoothie

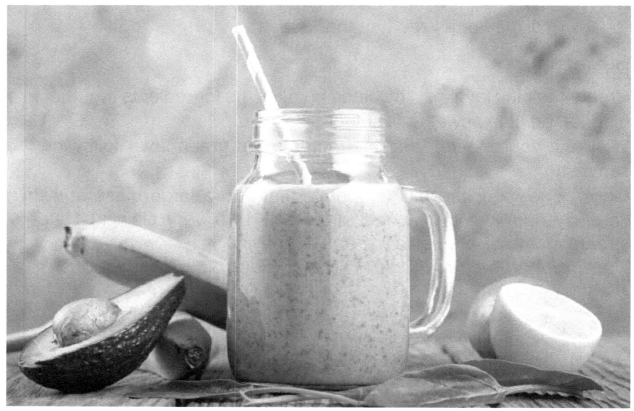

Prep Time: 1 minute

Cooking Time: 1 minute

Servings: 1 person

Tastes awesome and nutritious too! This smoothie is so thick that you would need to use a spoon. Feel free to add a tablespoon of pure honey to this smoothie. You can even top your glass with some shredded coconut and enjoy.

Ingredients

- ¼ cup almond milk, unsweetened
- A handful of fresh spinach
- ½ ripe avocado, small-sized
- 1 ripe banana, frozen
- ¼ teaspoon cinnamon
- ½ teaspoon vanilla

Directions

Blend all of the ingredients together in a blender, on high power until creamy.

Pour the mixture into a large glass, serve immediately and enjoy.

Nutritional Value: kcal: 284, Fat: 14 g, Fiber: 11 g, Protein: 5.1 g

Protein-Packed Green Smoothie

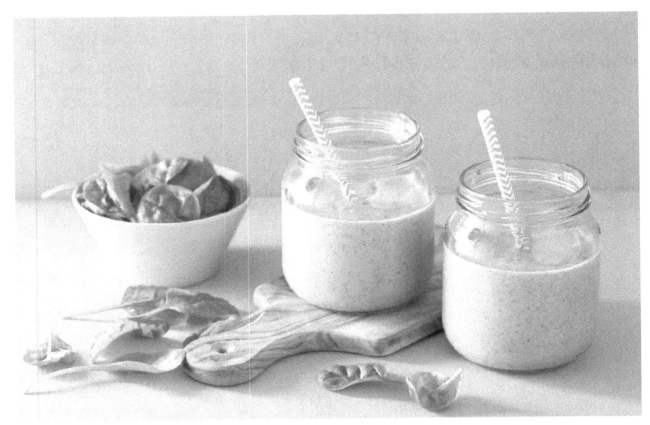

Prep Time: 20 minutes

Cooking Time: 40 minutes

Servings: 6 persons

If you prefer a sweeter smoothie, then sub the grapefruit juice with coconut water or even orange juice. For added protein, feel free to add half a scoop of your favorite protein powder.

<u>Ingredients</u>

- 1 sweet apple, large-sized, cored & chopped roughly
- ½ cup of red grapefruit juice, fresh
- 1 cup baby spinach or kale, fresh
- 2 tablespoons packed mint leaves, fresh
- 3 tablespoons hemp hearts, or to taste
- 1 celery stalk, medium to large-sized, chopped
- 1/3 cup mango, frozen

- 1 cup cucumber, chopped
- Ice cubes, as required
- Optional Ingredients:
- 1 ½ teaspoons virgin coconut oil

Directions

Add ½ cup of the fresh grapefruit juice to your blender.

Now add the spinach or kale followed by mango, hemp, apple, celery, cucumber, coconut oil, mint, and ice. Blend until completely smooth, on high power. Feel free to add some water, if required to blend the ingredients together.

Pour the mixture into a large glass, serve immediately and enjoy.

Nutritional Value: kcal: 196, Fat: 6 g, Fiber: 5 g, Protein: 6 g

Tropical Green Smoothie

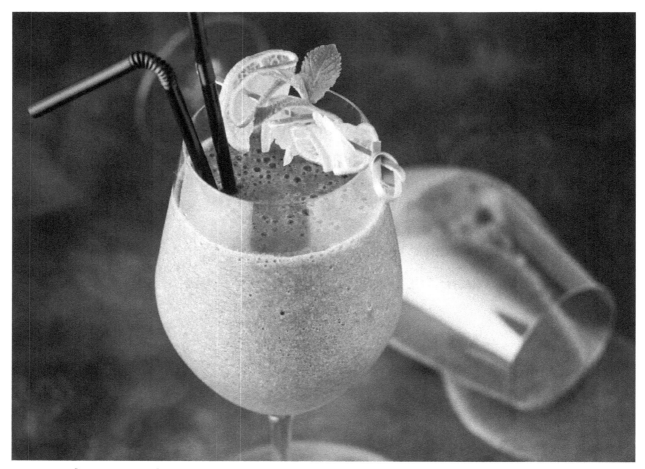

Prep Time: 1 minute

Cooking Time: 1 minute

Servings: 1 person

This recipe tastes very much similar to virgin piña colada. For added protein, feel free to add a dollop of yogurt and a scoop of your favorite protein powder. You can even top your smoothie with dried fruits and/or coconut flakes.

<u>Ingredients</u>

- 1 cup pineapple chunks, frozen
- 2 cups spinach, frozen
- 1 cup mixed berries such as blueberries, strawberries, raspberries
- 1 ripe banana, medium-sized, peeled, previously frozen

- 1 teaspoon vanilla extract
- 1 cup milk, any of your favorite
- Sweetener such as maple syrup, agave, sugar, Medjool dates, honey, stevia, as required, to taste
- 1 cup mango chunks, frozen

Directions

Place all of the ingredients together in a blender or Vita-Mix & blend until completely smooth & creamy, on high power. Serve immediately and enjoy.

Nutritional Value: kcal: 491, Fat: 6.5 g, Fiber: 12 g, Protein: 14 g

Green Smoothie with Blueberries & Peanut Butter

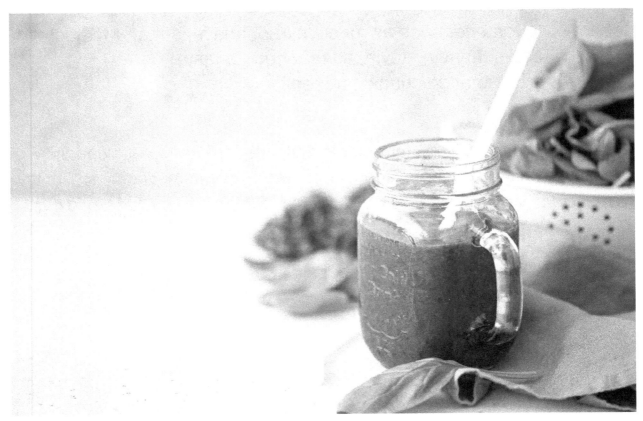

Prep Time: 1 minute

Cooking Time: 1 minute

Servings: 1 person

Absolutely delicious and a savior! If you want your drink to be a little thicker, then feel free to add more blueberries to your blender. You can use any of your favorite yogurts, such as plain, vanilla, or even blueberry, in this recipe.

Ingredients

- 1 ½ cups spinach, fresh
- 1 ripe banana, medium-sized
- ¼ cup yogurt
- 1 cup blueberries, frozen
- ½ tablespoon creamy peanut butter
- 1 tablespoon chia seeds

- A splash of milk, any of your favorite

Directions

Blend all of the ingredients together in a blender until completely smooth. Once done, add in the chia seeds & continue to pulse the ingredients for a couple of more times. Pour this mixture into a large glass, serve immediately & enjoy.

Nutritional Value: kcal: 335, Fat: 9 g, Fiber: 11 g, Protein: 9 g

Delicious Green Smoothie

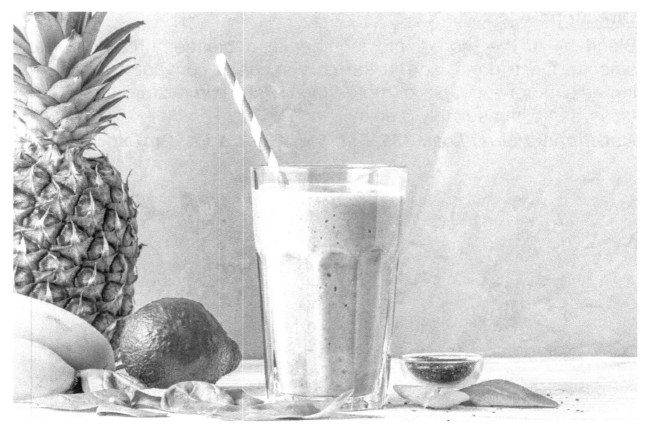

Prep Time: 1 minute

Cooking Time: 1 minute

Servings: 1 person

You should try this recipe when it's too hot outside. This smoothie is quite refreshing and packed with essential nutrients as well. Feel free to add sweetener to this smoothie if it's not sweet enough to your taste

Ingredients

- 2 cups fresh spinach
- 1 cup frozen pineapple chunks
- ½ ripe avocado
- 2 ½ cups almond milk
- 1 tablespoon chia seeds

Directions

Blend all of the ingredients together in a blender until completely smooth. Pour the mixture into a mason jar or cup. Serve immediately and enjoy.

Nutritional Value: kcal: 510, Fat: 22 g, Fiber: 14 g, Protein: 8.2 g

Matcha Pear Green Protein Smoothie

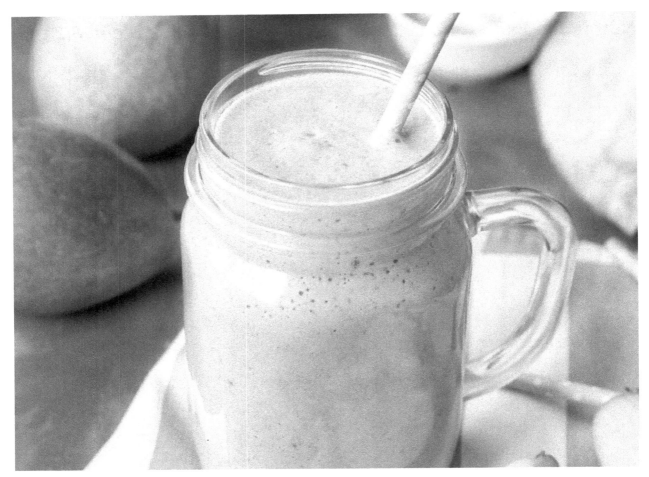

Prep Time: 1 minute

Cooking Time: 1 minute

Servings: 1 person

Feel free to top your drink with your favorite nuts and enjoy the taste. You can even top your drink with a handful of fresh blueberries.

Ingredients

- 1 pear, large-sized, cored
- 1 cup almond milk, unsweetened
- 1 scoop of Vanilla protein powder
- 1 cup fresh spinach
- ½ teaspoon Matcha tea powder

Directions

Combine all of the ingredients together in a blender until smooth and creamy, on high power. Fill a large glass with the prepared mixture. Serve immediately and enjoy.

Nutritional Value: kcal: 269, Fat: 8.8 g, Fiber: 11.6 g, Protein: 21 g

Spinach Orange Green Smoothie

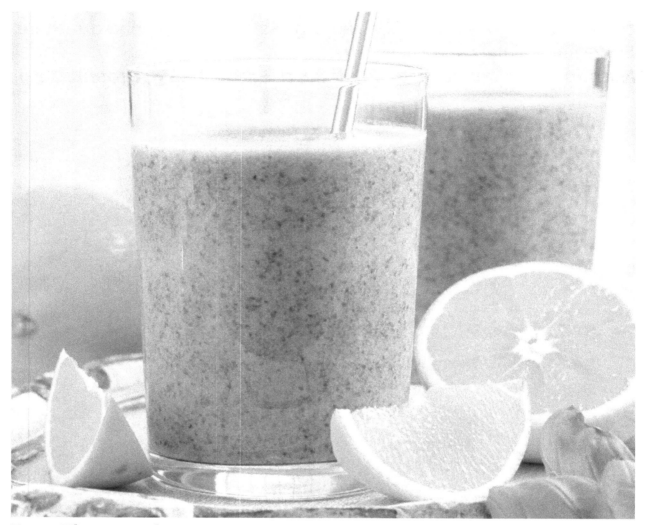

Prep Time: 1 minute

Cooking Time: 1 minute

Servings: 1 person

Absolutely delicious and healthy! You can even add a few apricots to this recipe.

<u>Ingredients</u>

- 1 cup organic spinach, tightly packed
- ½ ripe banana, peeled
- 1 navel orange, peeled
- ¼ cup coconut water

- Ice cubes, as required
- Optional Ingredients:
- 1 tablespoon hemp seeds

Directions

Add all of the ingredients with a few ice cubes into a blender, blend until combined well, on high power.

Feel free to add more of coconut water until you get desired level of consistency. Pour into a large glass, serve immediately & enjoy.

Nutritional Value: kcal: 189, Fat: 4.2 g, Fiber: 6.1 g, Protein: 6.1 g

Orange Kale Protein Green Smoothie

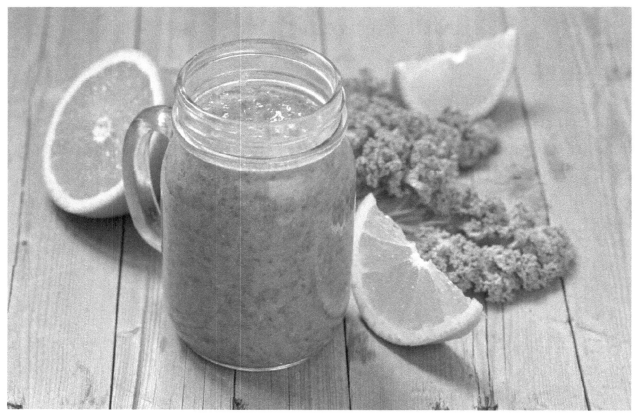

Prep Time: 1 minute

Cooking Time: 1 minute

Servings: 1 person

This smoothie recipe is packed with protein and nutrients. This smoothie would keep you satisfied for hours. You can sub the protein powder with plant-based protein powder and enjoy.

Ingredients

- 1 cup raw kale, chopped
- 2 scoops of vanilla protein powder
- 1 orange, peel & remove the seeds
- ½ teaspoon of spirulina powder
- 1 cup water
- A pinch each of ground cinnamon, and ginger powder

Directions

Combine all of the ingredients together in a blender until smooth and creamy, on high power. Serve immediately and enjoy.

Nutritional Value: kcal: 222, Fat: 1.1 g, Fiber: 3.1 g, Protein: 46 g

Super Healthy Green Smoothie

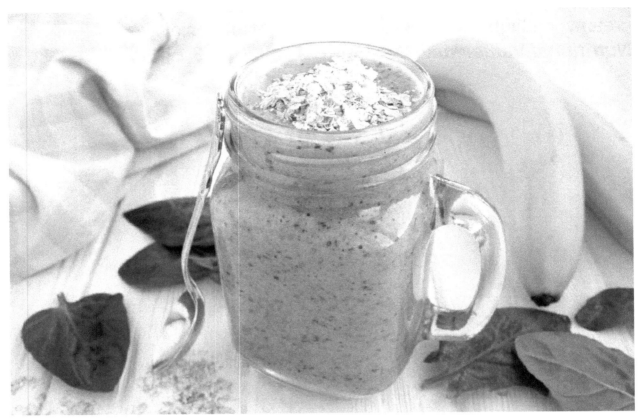

Prep Time: 2 minutes

Cooking Time: 2 minutes

Servings: 1 person

This smoothie is very thick and healthy. A nice way to consume some greens into your daily routine! Feel free to sprinkle your drink with the ancient granola and enjoy the taste.

Ingredients

- ½ ripe banana, large-sized
- ¼ cup rolled oats, raw
- 2 large handfuls of fresh spinach
- ¾ cup any of your favorite milk
- 1 tablespoon flax
- ½ scoop of Vega Choc-a-Lot

Directions

Combine all of the ingredients together in a blender until smooth and creamy, on high power. Serve immediately and enjoy.

Nutritional Value: kcal: 284, Fat: 7.6 g, Fiber: 7.2 g, Protein: 11 g

Sweet Honeydew Mint Smoothie

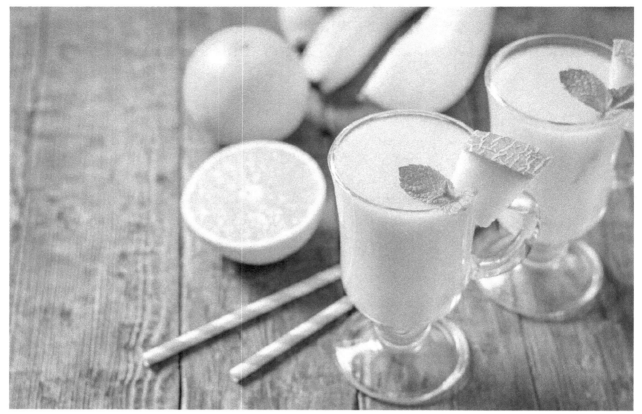

Prep Time: 2 minutes

Cooking Time: 2 minutes

Servings: 4 persons

This smoothie is perfect for a hot summer day. Just refresh your day with this drink and enjoy the taste. Just before serving, don't forget to garnish your drink with fresh mint leaves, you can also garnish your glass with fresh slices of melon.

Ingredients

- 4 cups honeydew melon, cut into small chunks (roughly 1 ½ pounds)
- 1 cup ice
- ½ to 1 teaspoon lime juice, fresh or to taste
- Fresh mint, leaves, plus more for garnish
- ½ cup coconut milk, light

- Drizzle of coconut nectar or honey, to taste

Directions

Remove the seeds from your melon, slice the outer rind away then, cut into small chunks.

Once done, add the melon chunks along with the lime, mint, coconut milk, and ice to the blender. Blend on high power until completely smooth.

Taste & adjust the amount of sweetness with coconut nectar or pure honey.

Serve immediately and enjoy.

Nutritional Value: kcal: 94, Fat: 2.2 g, Fiber: 1.3 g, Protein: 1.0 g

Peachy Green Protein Smoothie

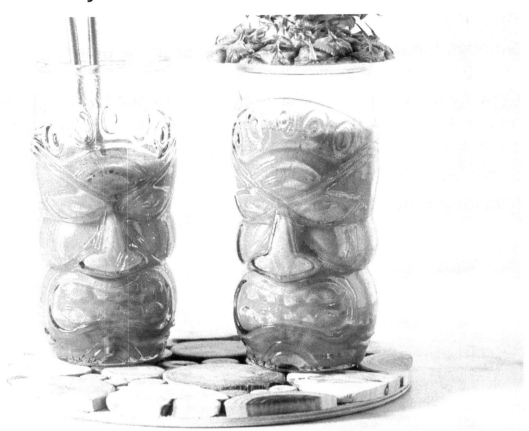

Prep Time: 2 minutes

Cooking Time: 2 minutes

Servings: 1 person

Enjoy this smoothie, the first thing in the morning. This smoothie would give you enough strength and energy throughout the day.

<u>Ingredients</u>

- ½ cup pineapple, frozen
- 2 cups of fresh kale
- 1 cup almond milk, unsweetened
- 2 scoops of Fuel-6 in vanilla, preferably daily burn
- 1 cup peaches, frozen
- ½ ripe banana, large-sized
- 1 tablespoon ground flaxseed

Directions

Add all of the ingredients together in a blender and blend on high power until mixed well. Serve immediately and enjoy.

Nutritional Value: kcal: 326, Fat: 7.2 g, Fiber: 7.1 g, Protein: 6.1 g

Hyper Monkey Blended Smoothie

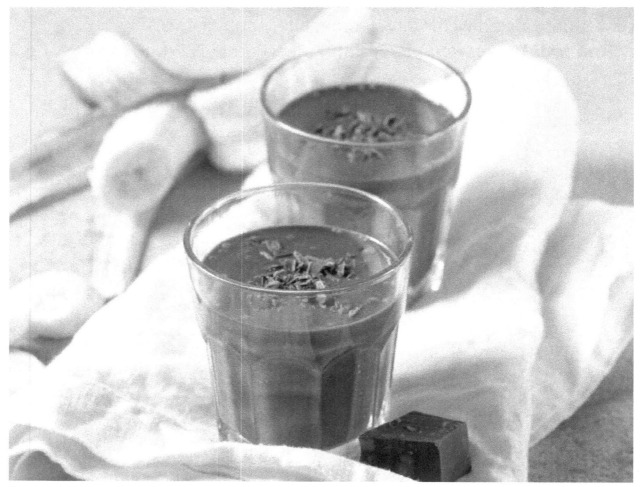

Prep Time: 2 minutes

Cooking Time: 2 minutes

Servings: 2 persons

This smoothie recipe is quite easy to prepare and full of flavors. Once you try this smoothie, I am sure you would prepare it again and would simply avoid having any other smoothies. Feel free to sweeten your drink with a bit of agave syrup, if required.

Ingredients

- ¼ cup slightly cooled strong espresso
- ¾ cup whole milk
- ¼ cup dark chocolate, chopped roughly

- ½ cup banana slices, frozen
- ¼ cup peanut butter, smooth
- Ice, as required

Directions

Pour espresso and milk into a blender and then, add in the peanut butter and frozen banana. Add approximately half a cup of the ice. Cover & blend until smooth, on high power.

Next, add in the chopped dark chocolate & pulse again until chocolate bits are nicely distributed, for a few more seconds.

Serve immediately, garnished with more of chocolate chunks and a banana slice.

Nutritional Value: kcal: 430, Fat: 24 g, Fiber: 4 g, Protein: 11 g

Happy Green Monster Smoothie

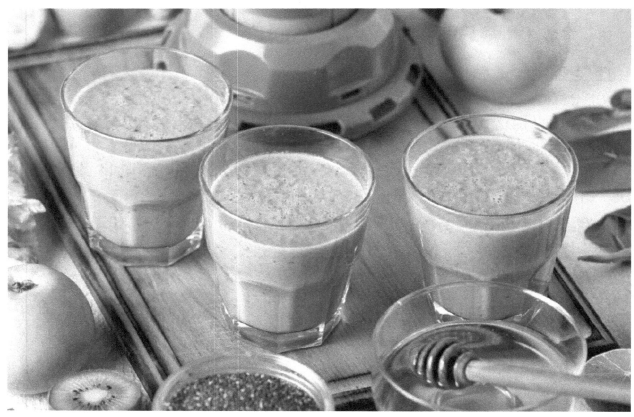

Prep Time: 2 minutes

Cooking Time: 2 minutes

Servings: 2 persons

Absolutely delicious and healthy! You can even add kiwi, pineapple, apple, lemon, and carrots to make this smoothie more nutritious.

Ingredients

- 1 pear, peeled and cored
- 2 handfuls of fresh spinach
- 1 tablespoon agave syrup
- Juice of half a lime, fresh
- 1/3 cup coconut milk
- 2 handfuls of fresh kale
- 1 cup coconut water

Directions

Pour coconut milk with coconut water & agave syrup in a blender and then, add in the fresh lime juice. Add pear, kale and spinach. Cover & pulse on high power for half a minute to a minute.

Serve immediately and enjoy.

Nutritional Value: kcal: 172, Fat: 4.1 g, Fiber: 4.3 g, Protein: 3.6 g

Vanilla Matcha Protein Smoothie Recipe

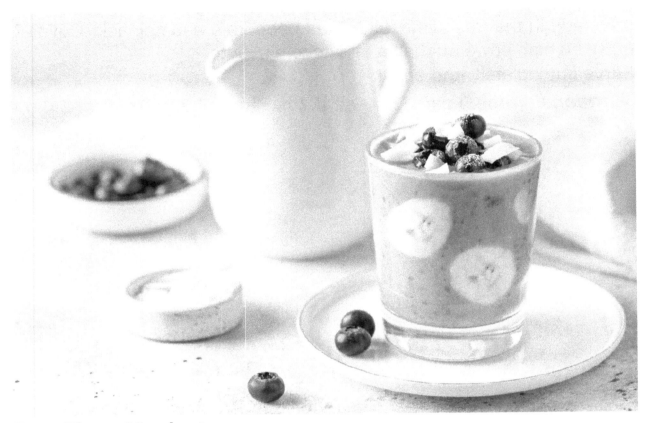

Prep Time: 10 minutes

Cooking Time: 1 hour & 10 minutes

Servings: 5 persons

We all enjoyed this wonderful smoothie recipe on the breakfast table. You can sub the almond milk with any of your favorite milk and enjoy it.

<u>Ingredients</u>

- 1 ripe banana, large-sized
- 2 scoops of vanilla protein powder
- ½ teaspoon maple syrup
- 2 teaspoons matcha green tea powder
- 1 cup almond milk, unsweetened
- Fresh vanilla bean, scraped from 1" of a pod
- ½ cup ice

Directions

Add all of the ingredients together in a blender and blend on high power until mixed well. Serve immediately and enjoy.

Nutritional Value: kcal: 376, Fat: 3 g, Fiber: 6.1 g, Protein: 5.2 g

Apple-Kale Green Smoothie Recipe

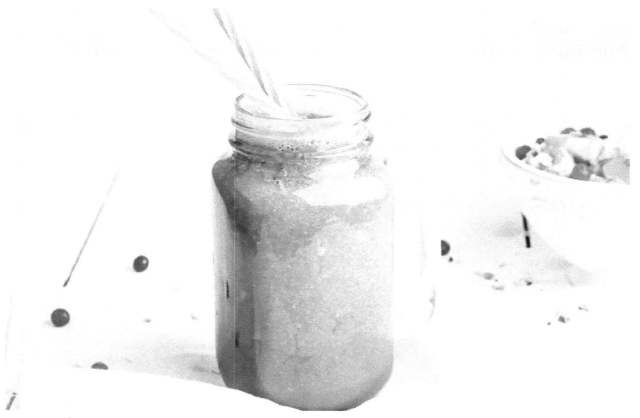

Prep Time: 10 minutes

Cooking Time: 30 minutes

Servings: 6 persons

You can use any of your favorite apples in this smoothie. If you don't have time for breakfast or running short of your time, this smoothie will keep you full till your next meal.

Ingredients

- 1 cup raw kale, chopped
- 1 cup almond milk, unsweetened
- 2 scoops (1 packet) DailyBurn Fuel-6 Protein in vanilla
- 1 green apple, small-sized, cored & chopped
- 1 small cucumber, chopped
- 1 teaspoon lemon juice, fresh

Directions

Add all of the ingredients together in a blender and blend on high power until mixed well. Serve immediately and enjoy.

Nutritional Value: kcal: 273, Fat: 4.2 g, Fiber: 6.8 g, Protein: 6.4 g

Summer Breezes Smoothie

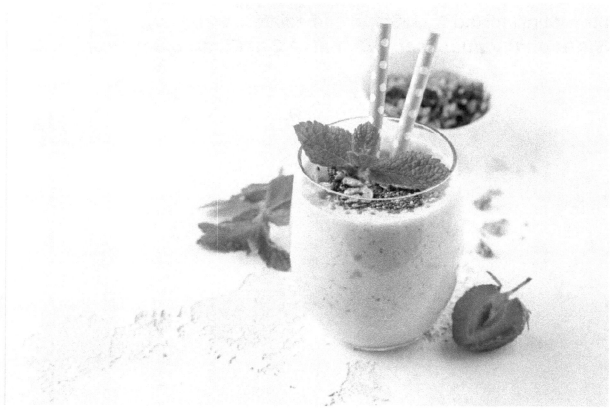

Prep Time: 10 minutes

Cooking Time: 10 minutes

Servings: 3 persons

Enjoy this delicious smoothie as a breakfast recipe. Feel free to add a few dates to this smoothie and just before serving, garnish your glass with a few fresh mint leaves, a pineapple slice, and a fresh strawberry.

Ingredients

- 1 cup canned pineapple, crushed, in juice
- 6 strawberries, medium-sized
- 1 cup plain yogurt, nonfat
- 1 banana, medium-sized
- 4 ice cubes
- 1 teaspoon vanilla extract

Directions

Combine all of the ingredients together in a blender until combined well, for a minute or two, on high power. Pour the mixture into a large glass, serve immediately and enjoy.

Nutritional Value: kcal: 121, Fat: 0.2 g, Fiber: 1.2 g, Protein: 4.6 g

Berries Packed Fruit Smoothie

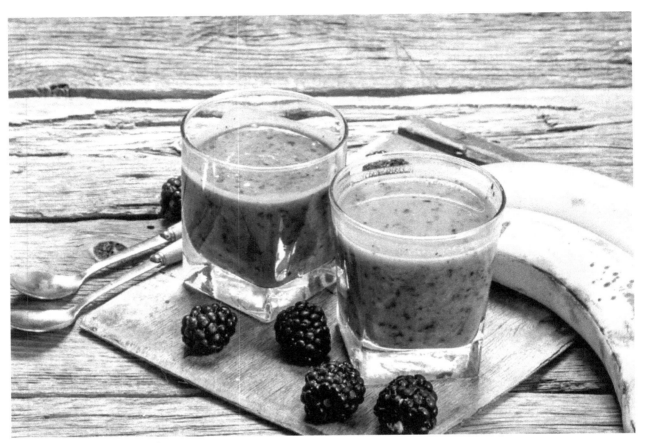

Prep Time: 2 minutes

Cooking Time: 2 minutes

Servings: 2 persons

I often prepare this smoothie recipe for my family members and serve it with blueberries on top. Feel free to serve your glass with a few chopped nuts as well.

Ingredients

- 1 cup blackberries, frozen, plus more for garnish
- 1 ¼ cup almond milk
- 1 ripe banana
- 1 cup raspberries, frozen
- ½ cup Greek yogurt
- 1 cup strawberries, frozen

Directions

Combine all of the ingredients together in a blender until combined well, for a minute or two, on high power. Evenly divide the mixture between two large glasses. Serve immediately, garnished with blackberries and enjoy.

Nutritional Value: kcal: 112, Fat: 2.8 g, Fiber: 2.2 g, Protein: 4.4 g

Delicious Banana Smoothie

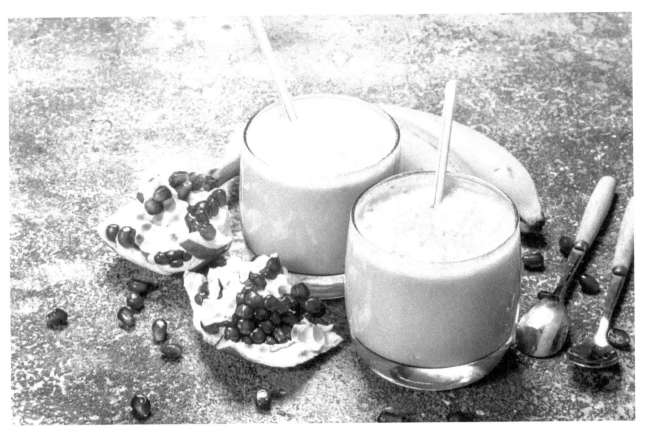

Prep Time: 20 minutes

Cooking Time: 1 hour & 30 minutes

Servings: 8 persons

This recipe is very famous in India. It's also known as banana shake. Feel free to use almond milk in this smoothie. Absolutely delicious and healthy. Rather than adding the cinnamon powder, you can add ¼ teaspoon of vanilla powder or extract as well.

Ingredients

- ½ cup coconut milk
- 3 ripe bananas, large-sized
- Toasted seeds & nuts for garnish
- ¼ teaspoon cinnamon powder

Directions

Peel three bananas, chop and add the pieces into a blender.

Next, add ½ cup coconut milk and ¼ teaspoon cinnamon powder.

Blend on high power until completely smooth. Once done, pour the mixture in a large-sized serving glass.

Serve immediately, garnished with toasted nuts and seeds, enjoy.

Nutritional Value: kcal: 127, Fat: 8.5 g, Fiber: 2.7 g, Protein: 2.3 g

Strawberry Banana Smoothie

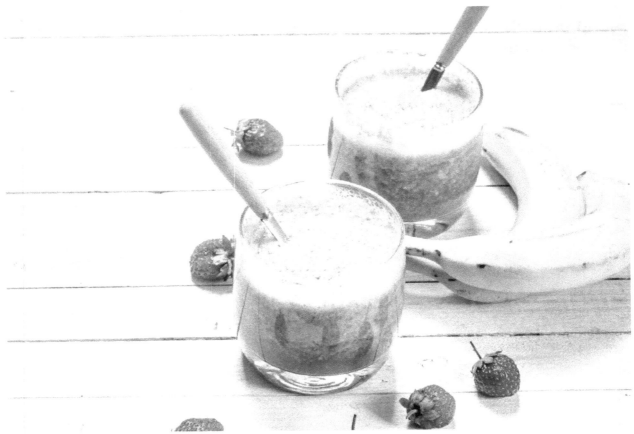

Prep Time: 20 minutes

Cooking Time: 40 minutes

Servings: 2 persons

Absolutely delicious, nutritious, refreshing and healthy smoothie! Feel free to add a handful of fresh mint or basil to your drink. You can sub the almond milk with oat milk and can sub honey with maple syrup as well.

Ingredients

- 1 cup strawberries
- 1 ½ cups raspberries
- 1 tablespoon pure honey
- ½ banana, frozen
- 1 cup almond milk
- 1 ½ cups ice

Directions

Combine all of the ingredients together in a blender until combined well, for a minute or two, on high power. Evenly divide the mixture between two large glasses

Taste and add ½ cup of more almond milk and one tablespoon of more honey if it's too tart. Serve immediately and enjoy.

Nutritional Value: kcal: 121, Fat: 4 g, Fiber: 3.1 g, Protein: 4.4 g

Fruit & Yogurt Smoothie

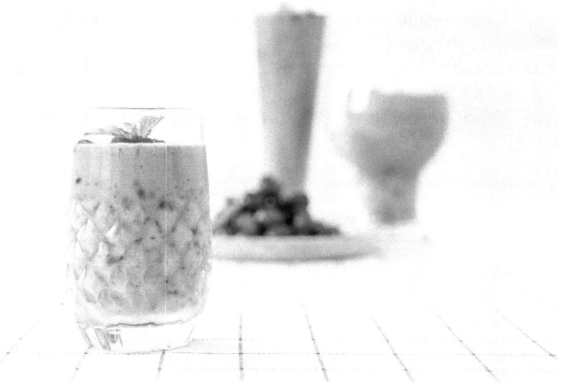

Prep Time: 2 minutes
Cooking Time: 2 minutes
Servings: 2 persons

You can use tofu instead of yogurt and can add a few pecans and almonds. You can also add milk instead of the fruit juice. Let's try it!

Ingredients

- 1 ½ cups frozen fruit like, raspberries, blueberries, peaches or pineapple
- ¾ cup plain yogurt, nonfat
- ½ cup fruit juice, 100% pure

Directions

Puree juice with yogurt in a blender for a minute, until completely smooth. With the motor still running, slowly add in the fruit & continue to puree until the mixture is completely smooth.

Nutritional Value: kcal: 276, Fat: 3.2 g, Fiber: 4.4 g, Protein: 11.2 g

Unicorn Smoothie

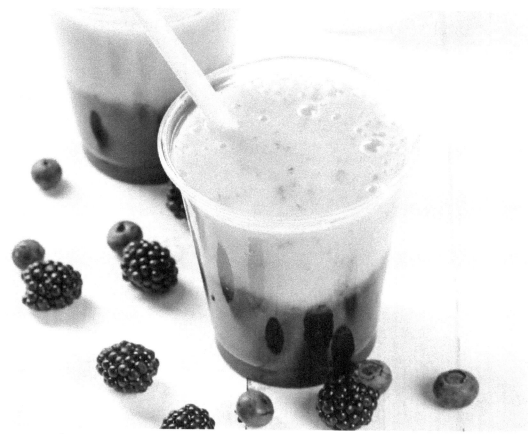

Prep Time: 10 minutes

Cooking Time: 10 minutes

Servings: 4 persons

My entire family is just crazy about this delicious smoothie recipe. They often ask me to prepare it for them for breakfast. Garnish your glass with kiwi, star fruit, mixed berries, and chia seeds tied on wooden skewers.

Ingredients

- 1 ½ cups vanilla yogurt, low-fat, divided
- 1 cup frozen blueberries or blackberries
- 1 ½ cups low-fat milk, divided
- 1 cup mango chunks, frozen
- 3 ripe bananas, large, divided
- 1 cup strawberries or raspberries, frozen

Directions

Combine all of the ingredients together in a blender and blend on high power until smooth and creamy. Pour the mixture among four glasses. Serve and enjoy.

Nutritional Value: kcal: 252, Fat: 1.7 g, Fiber: 6 g, Protein: 9.2 g

Nutriboost Smoothie

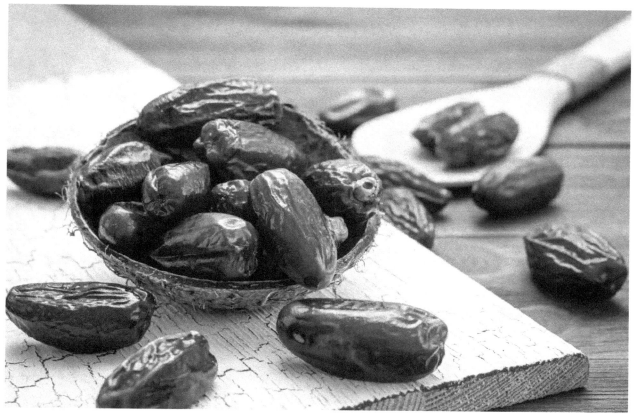

Prep Time: 10 minutes

Cooking Time: 10 minutes

Servings: 2 persons

Absolutely delicious and surely a keeper! This smoothie is low in calories, rich in potassium, iron, antioxidants, and magnesium.

Ingredients

- ¼ cup dates, chopped into small pieces
- 1 banana, medium-sized, chopped into small pieces
- ¾ cup almond milk

Directions

Combine all of the ingredients in a blender until completely smooth & creamy. Fill two glasses evenly with the prepared mixture. Serve and enjoy.

Nutritional Value: kcal: 120, Fat: 2 g, Fiber: 4.1 g, Protein: 4 g

Birthday Cake Smoothie

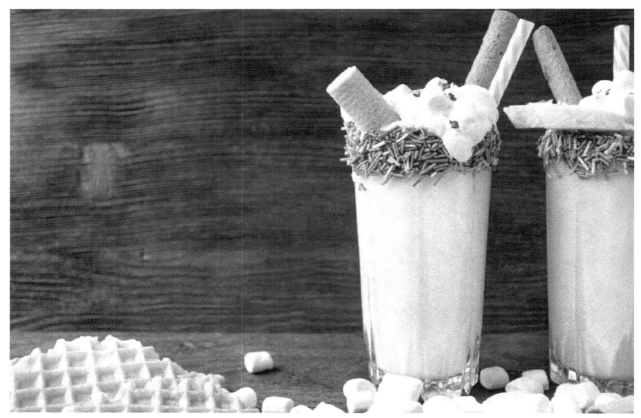

Prep Time: 20 minutes

Cooking Time: 40 minutes

Servings: 6 persons

This smoothie tastes more like a cake batter and is a healthy choice too. Feel free to top your drink with some whipped cream and then top with the sprinkles. Enjoy.

Ingredients

- 1 cup cashew milk
- ¼ cup rolled oats
- 1 banana frozen
- A scoop of vanilla protein powder
- 1 teaspoon vanilla extract
- 1 tablespoon sprinkles

Directions

Combine all of the ingredients in a blender until completely smooth & creamy. Fill a glass with the prepared mixture. Serve immediately, garnished with the sprinkles and enjoy.

Nutritional Value: kcal: 224, Fat: 4 g, Fiber: 2.4 g, Protein: 4 g

Pecan Pie Smoothie

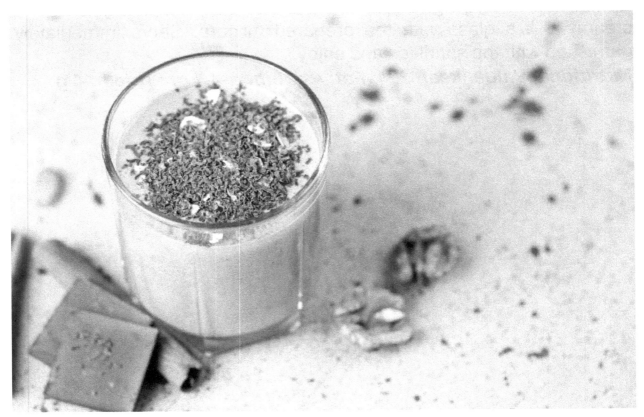

Prep Time: 2 minutes

Cooking Time: 2 minutes

Servings: 2 persons

This is one of my favorite vegan smoothies. Don't forget to soak the pecans and medjool dates in water for half an hour.

Ingredients

- ¼ cup pecans
- ½ teaspoon vanilla extract
- 2 Medjool dates
- ¾ teaspoon cinnamon
- 1½ cups almond milk
- ½ cup ice cubes
- Coconut whipped cream, as required, to top

Directions

Combine all of the ingredients together in a blender until completely smooth.
Serve immediately, topped with the coconut whipped cream and enjoy.
Nutritional Value: kcal: 214, Fat: 7 g, Fiber: 4 g, Protein: 6 g

Galaxy Smoothie

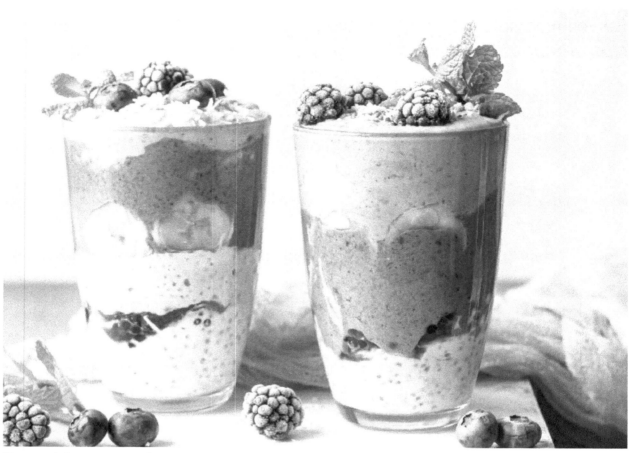

Prep Time: 2 minutes

Cooking Time: 2 minutes

Servings: 1 person

You would fall in love with this smoothie recipe. Feel free to create a layer of whipped cream on top and then sprinkle with your favorite nuts.

Ingredients

- 1 cup cashew milk
- 1 banana, frozen
- 1 cup coconut yogurt
- 1 teaspoon chia seeds
- 1 cup fresh blueberries

Directions

Add all of the ingredients (except 1 tablespoon coconut yogurt) to a blender, pulse on high power until smooth.

Next, create the galaxy look by pouring the reserved coconut yogurt in a glass, swirl around the inner edges.

Fill the prepared glass with the smoothie, serve and enjoy.

Nutritional Value: kcal: 382, Fat: 12 g, Fiber: 4 g, Protein: 6 g

Red Velvet Smoothie

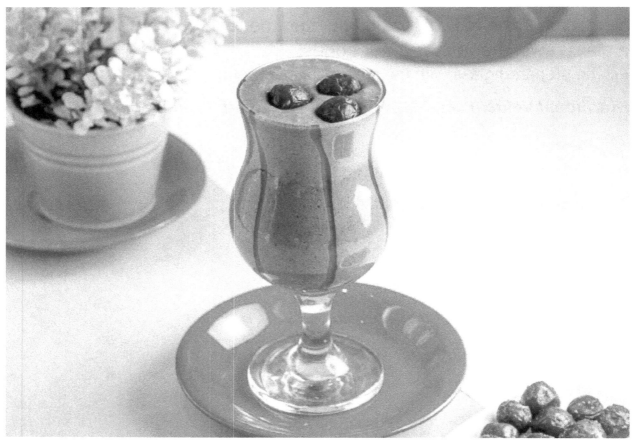

Prep Time: 2 minutes

Cooking Time: 2 minutes

Servings: 1 person

This smoothie tastes more like a chocolate and is surely a keeper. For more nutrition, feel free to add one teaspoon of beetroot powder and enjoy.

Ingredients

- 1 cup cherries, frozen
- ½ teaspoon vanilla extract
- 1 cup strawberries, frozen
- 1 ½ cups oat milk
- 1 tablespoon cocoa powder

Directions

Combine all of the ingredients together in a blender, blend on high power until completely smooth and creamy. Pour into a large-sized serving glass and enjoy

Nutritional Value: kcal: 368, Fat: 2 g, Fiber: 4 g, Protein: 3 g

Peanut Butter Cup Smoothie

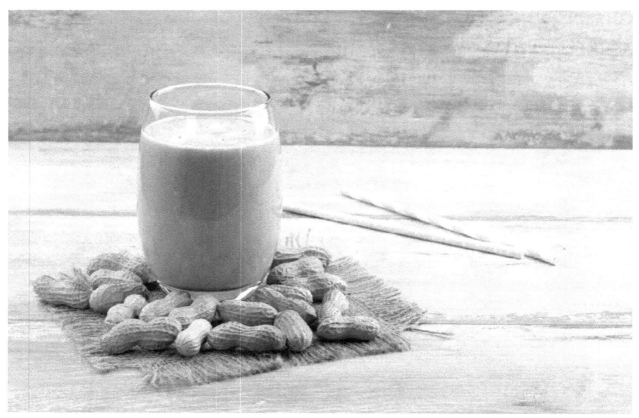

Prep Time: 2 minutes

Cooking Time: 2 minutes

Servings: 1 person

This smoothie is packed with essential nutrients and antioxidants. Feel free to sprinkle your favorite nuts on top and enjoy.

Ingredients

- 2 tablespoons peanut butter
- 1 cup banana, frozen
- 2 tablespoon rolled oats
- ¼ cup plant milk
- 2 tablespoons cocoa powder

Directions

Combine all of the ingredients together in a blender, blend on high power until completely smooth and creamy. Pour into a large-sized serving glass and enjoy

Nutritional Value: kcal: 222, Fat: 7.7 g, Fiber: 6 g, Protein: 4 g

Apple Banana Smoothie

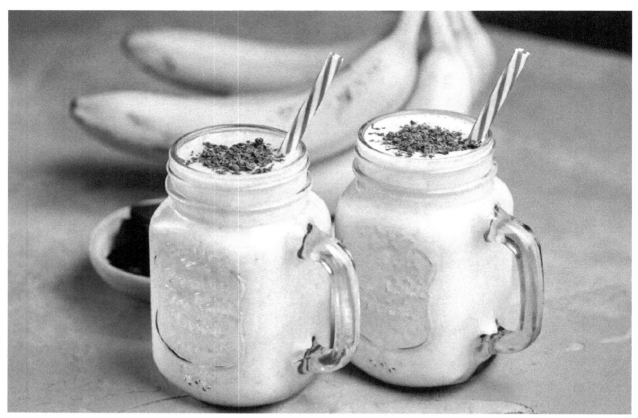

Prep Time: 2 minutes

Cooking Time: 2 minutes

Servings: 2 persons

Cacao nibs are optional in this smoothie but it surely enhances the tastes. Feel free to serve this smoothie with chopped banana and granola.

Ingredients

- 1 apple, peeled & chopped
- 6 to 7 dates, chopped
- 1 banana, ripe, large, chopped
- 1 ½ cups whole milk
- 1 to 2 teaspoons cacao nibs

Directions

Combine all of the ingredients together in a blender, blend on high power until completely smooth and creamy. Pour into a large-sized serving glass and enjoy.

Nutritional Value: kcal: 260, Fat: 4 g, Fiber: 4 g, Protein: 6 g

Oatmeal Smoothie

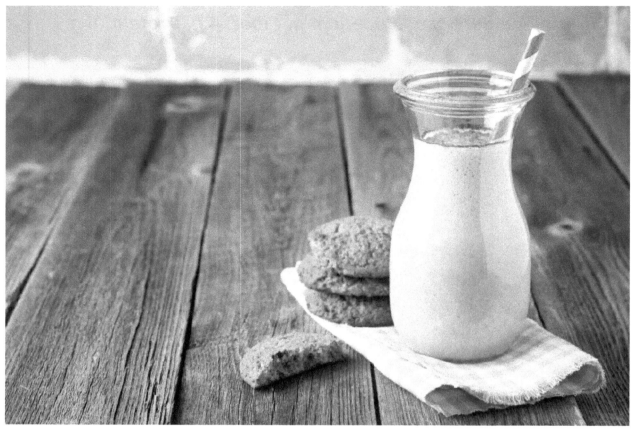

Prep Time: 2 minutes

Cooking Time: 2 minutes

Servings: 1 person

This delicious smoothie recipe is very delicious and easy to digest. It's packed with fiber, healthy fats, and protein. Feel free to add ice at the end if you are looking for a thicker smoothie.

Ingredients

- ½ teaspoon pure vanilla extract
- ¼ cup quick oats or old-fashioned oats
- ½ cup almond milk, unsweetened
- 1 banana, frozen and chopped into small chunks
- ½ tablespoon pure maple syrup plus more to taste
- 1 tablespoon creamy peanut butter

- 1/8 teaspoon kosher salt
- ½ teaspoon ground cinnamon

Directions

Pulse the oats in a blender until ground finely. Once done, add in the banana, maple syrup, peanut butter, milk, cinnamon, vanilla, and salt. Continue to blend the ingredients until completely smooth & creamy, stopping & scrapping the sides of your blender down, as required. Taste & add more of sweetener, if required. Serve immediately & enjoy.

Nutritional Value: kcal: 317, Fat: 10 g, Fiber: 6 g, Protein: 7 g

Almond Fruit Smoothie

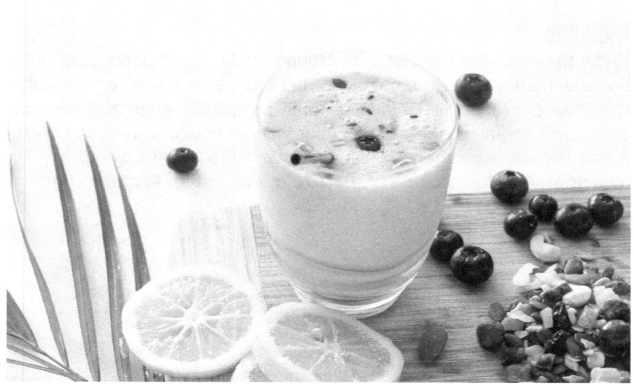

Prep Time: 2 minutes

Cooking Time: 2 minutes

Servings: 2 persons

A perfect vegan option that you can serve to your guests! Feel free to garnish your glasses with mango slices and enjoy.

Ingredients

- 2 tablespoons slivered almonds, toasted
- 1 cup frozen peaches
- 2 cups orange juice
- 1 banana, frozen, peeled & chopped

Directions

First, blend the peaches with banana in a blender until smooth.

Once done, immediately add & blend the orange juice

Pour the mixture evenly into two large glasses. Serve immediately, topped with toasted almonds and enjoy.

Nutritional Value: kcal: 222, Fat: 6 g, Fiber: 4 g, Protein: 6 g

Detox Smoothie

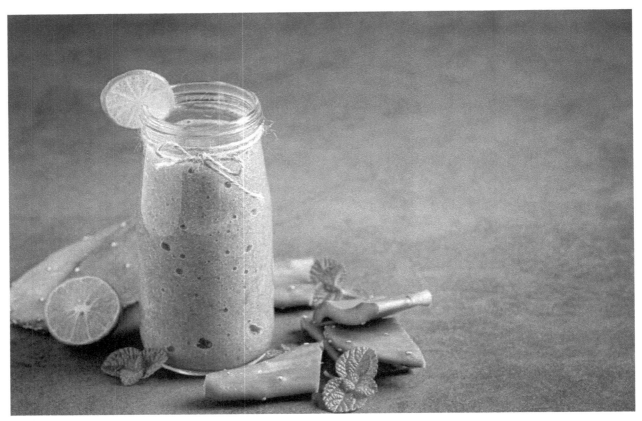

Prep Time: 2 minutes

Cooking Time: 2 minutes

Servings: 2 persons

My grandmother used to prepare this smoothie for us. For added nutrition, feel free to add 1/8 teaspoon finely grated lemon zest and ¼ cup frozen raw broccoli.

Ingredients

- 1 cup filtered water or raw coconut water, plus more as required
- 1 tablespoon lemon juice, fresh
- 1 green apple, medium-sized, skin on, cored & diced
- 1 cup baby spinach
- 1 small red beet, raw, peeled & diced
- 1 cup strawberries, frozen
- ½ small avocado, pitted & peeled

- 1 cup pineapple, frozen
- A pinch of cayenne pepper

Directions

Combine all of the ingredients together in a blender, blend on high power for a minute, until completely smooth. Pour the mixture into a large glass, serve immediately & enjoy.

Nutritional Value: kcal: 161, Fat: 6 g, Fiber: 3 g, Protein: 4 g

Fruit and Milk Smoothie

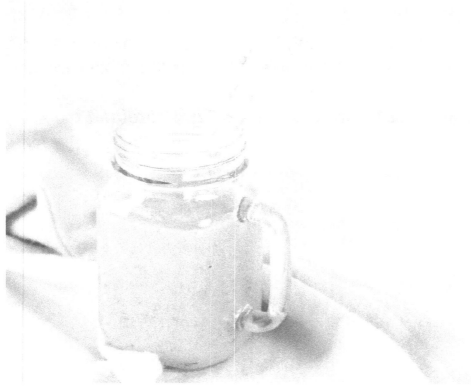

Prep Time: 2 minutes

Cooking Time: 2 minutes

Servings: 4 persons

Just before serving, garnish your glass with a slice of star fruit and enjoy.

Ingredients

- 1 cup unsweetened peaches, sliced, frozen
- 2 cups milk, preferably 2%
- 1 cup unsweetened strawberries, frozen
- 2 tablespoons honey
- ¼ cup orange juice, fresh

Directions

Combine all of the ingredients together in a blender. Cover & blend on high power until completely smooth. Pour the mixture into chilled glasses, serve immediately and enjoy.

Nutritional Value: kcal: 120, Fat: 2 g, Fiber: 1 g, Protein: 4 g

Pomegranate Smoothie

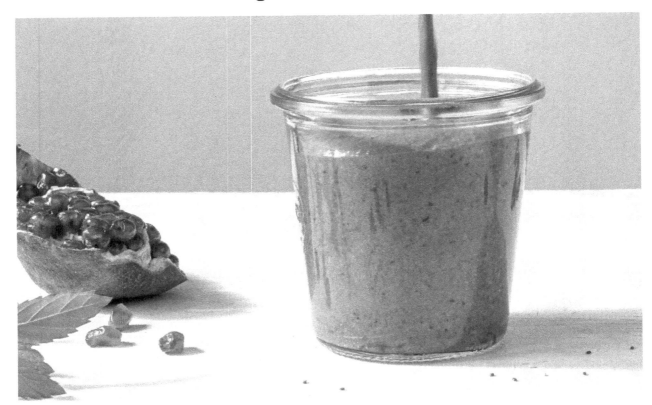

Prep Time: 2 minutes
Cooking Time: 2 minutes
Servings: 1 person

Just before serving, top your drink with pomegranate seeds. Feel free to add more milk or sweetener.

Ingredients

- 1 cup strawberries
- 2 cups orange juice, fresh
- ½ cup Greek yogurt
- 1 ripe banana, large-sized
- ½ cup pomegranate arils plus extra for serving

Directions

Combine all of the ingredients together in a blender, blend on high power until completely smooth and creamy.

Nutritional Value: kcal: 112, Fat: 6 g, Fiber: 4 g, Protein: 4.2 g

Grapefruit Ginger Smoothie

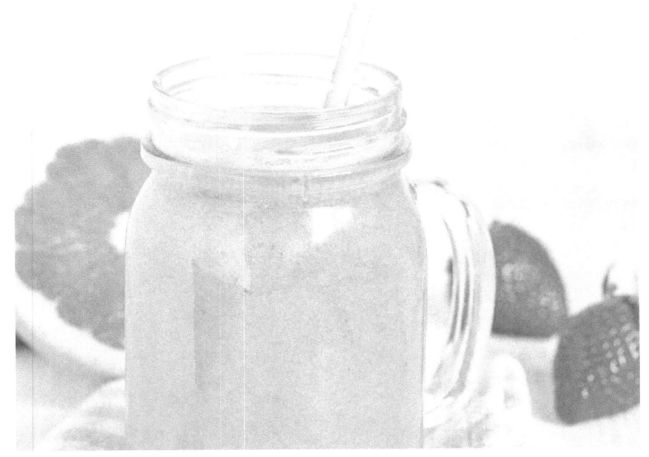

Prep Time: 2 minutes

Cooking Time: 2 minutes

Servings: 1 person

For a vegan version, use plant-based milk or coconut yogurt. Good for type II diabetic patients. Serve immediately and enjoy.

Ingredients

- 1 cup probiotic yogurt
- 1 large pink grapefruit, peeled, remove the bitter inner skin & seeds, reserve the segments
- 2" fresh ginger
- 1 medium carrot, peeled
- 3 to 4 Medjool dates or to taste

- 1 tablespoon maca powder
- Chia seeds for topping

Directions

Pulse all of the ingredients together in a blender until completely smooth, on high power.

Nutritional Value: kcal: 140, Fat: 4 g, Fiber: 2 g, Protein: 4 g

Grapefruit Juice Smoothie

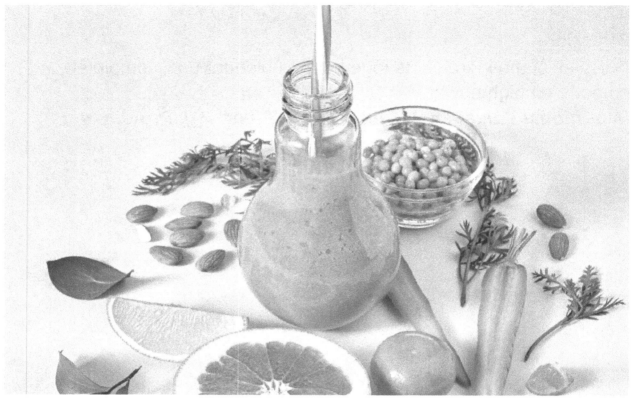

Prep Time: 2 minutes

Cooking Time: 2 minutes

Servings: 2 persons

You can even use vanilla yogurt in this recipe. Feel free to top your drink with a fresh strawberry and enjoy.

Ingredients

- 8 strawberries, large
- 1 ⅓ cups red grapefruit juice, fresh
- 2 tablespoons honey
- 1 container banana-strawberry yogurt (8-ounce)
- 2 medium bananas, sliced
- 1 cup ice, crushed

Directions

Pulse all of the ingredients together in a blender until completely smooth, on high power. Evenly divide the prepared mixture between two glasses. Serve immediately and enjoy.

Nutritional Value: kcal: 341, Fat: 2 g, Fiber: 3.1 g, Protein: 6.2 g

Banana Cinnamon Roll Smoothie

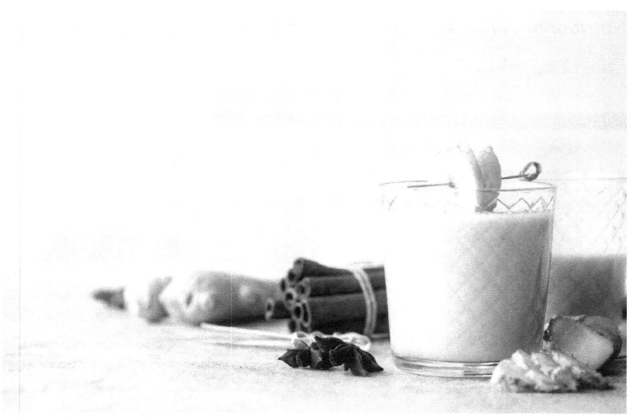

Prep Time: 2 minutes

Cooking Time: 2 minutes

Servings: 2 persons

Feel free to add coffee and protein powder to taste. Just before serving, add a few banana chunks and sprinkle with the cinnamon powder.

Ingredients

- 1 banana, frozen & broken into 4 pieces
- ¼ cup old fashioned oats
- 3 pitted medjool dates
- 1 teaspoon chia seeds
- ½ teaspoon ground cinnamon
- 1 teaspoon pure vanilla essence
- ½ cup Greek yogurt
- 1 cup almond milk

- 2-3 ice cubes

Directions

Pulse all of the ingredients together in a blender until completely smooth, on high power. Evenly divide the prepared mixture between two glasses. Serve immediately and enjoy.

Nutritional Value: kcal: 380, Fat: 16 g, Fiber: 2.5 g, Protein: 24 g

Tropical Smoothie

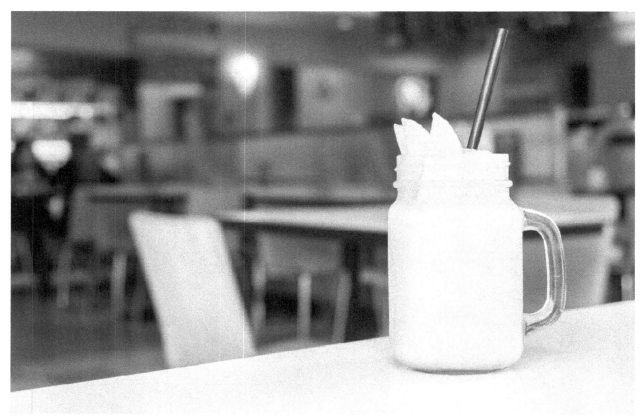

Prep Time: 5 minutes

Cooking Time: 5 minutes

Servings: 2 persons

This smoothie recipe is a keeper. Feel free to garnish your drink with ingredients such as raspberries, lime slices, and pineapple wedges. Rather than using the pineapple juice, you can use coconut water as well.

Ingredients

- 1 banana
- ¾ cup pineapple juice
- 1 cup mango, frozen
- A scoop of whey protein
- 1 cup pineapple, frozen
- ½ cup light coconut milk

Directions

Pulse all of the ingredients together in a blender for a minute, until completely smooth, on high power. Fill two large glasses with the prepared mixture. Serve immediately and enjoy.

Nutritional Value: kcal: 249, Fat: 12 g, Fiber: 10 g, Protein: 12 g

Pineapple Smoothie

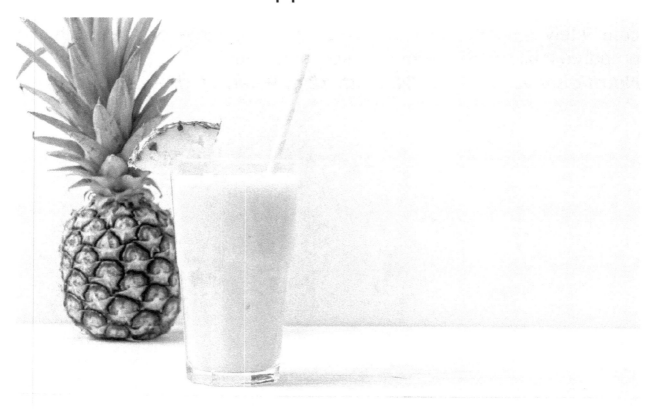

Prep Time: 2 minutes

Cooking Time: 2 minutes

Servings: 1 person

While blending, feel free to add a bit of water, if required, until you get your desired level of consistency. You can even prepare popsicles with this smoothie.

Ingredients

- ½ cup full-fat coconut milk, canned
- 1 cup frozen pineapple, cut into 1" pieces
- ½ cup orange juice
- ½ frozen banana, cut into coins

Directions

Combine all of the ingredients in a blender in the sequence mentioned above. Blend on high power until smooth and creamy. Serve immediately and enjoy.

Nutritional Value: kcal: 240, Fat: 10 g, Fiber: 7.2 g, Protein: 12 g

Conclusion

Thank you again for choosing this book.

With this book, you can get plenty of options to prepare smoothie recipes. Smoothie recipes are famous worldwide and these recipes don't need any special ingredient.

You can surprise your kiddos and your family just by preparing their favorite smoothie recipe for a special weekend breakfast.

With these smoothie recipes, your body would naturally get essential vitamins and minerals. Your body would get enough of antioxidants through fresh raw vegetables and fruits.

What are you still waiting for? If you haven't bought this book yet, then do it now, turn the pages, and surprise your family with your smoothie-making techniques.

Author's Afterthoughts

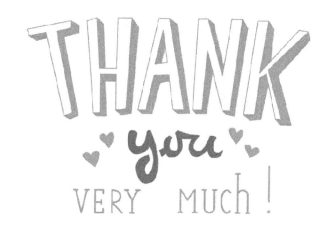

CPSIA information can be obtained
at www.ICGtesting.com
Printed in the USA
BVHW061056230621
610291BV00003B/286